The Plain Truth About Good Health

Six Simple Secrets to Radiant Health

Sparkle C. Duncan

DISCLAIMER

Sparkle C. Duncan is a health coach and health advocate, not a doctor, not a dietician and not a nutritionist. The Sparkle Lifestyle is not a health care provider, adviser or consultant. All content herein is the sole opinion of the author and in no way is intended to be or should be construed as medical advice or treatment. The reader or hearer of this information is solely responsible for his or her actions and the consequences thereof. If you want, need or seek medical advice or treatment, see a doctor.

CONTENTS

SPECIAL BONUS

ACKNOWLEDGMENTS

To my best friend who I've learned to lean on and fully trust although it's taken many years for me to get to this point, my Lord Jesus Christ. You have proven yourself to be truthful, loyal and trustworthy. At times when it felt like you were not around, you were there because whenever I fell, you always caught me before I hit the ground. I love you.

To my second best friend, my mother who has always believed in me, encouraged me and supported all of my endeavors with never a discouraging word. My mother is also the person who inspired me to write this book. As I searched for answers to the cause of her illnesses and ways to stop her decline without medicine, I realized that others were in need of this information as well.

To my father who I'm sure was the greatest contributor to my sense of humor. Thank you for working hard on your job, never missing a day and for being present when other fathers in our neighborhood were absent. Rest in peace Pop, I miss you.

To my acupuncturist and friend, Laila Nabulsi. Thank you for your support through some tough and scary times. Your wisdom, knowledge and skillful techniques for healing are amazing!

To my editor Laura Urista. Thank you so much for your assistance. Your help gave me the boost I needed to move forward.

To Bryan Tarr, my business coach and computer tech guy who continued to support me even when the money wasn't there. Thank you Bryan for your patience, encouragement and belief in me.

To Jerome Johnson. Thank you for your guidance and personal support and for quickly answering my texts or picking up the phone whenever I called. Thank you for your savvy and for your friendship.

To Donna Graham for the hours spent on the phone faithfully every morning for months at 7:00 a.m. Thank you for sharing your spiritual knowledge and equipping me for the struggles ahead. How did you know that there would be a strong presence determined to block my progress and the blessings of others through my work. You may be totally blind, but you have more insight than anyone I know.

To Les Brown. Thank you for encouraging me to pursue my goals and for reminding me that you began your career in the same manner that I started mine-by helping others with their issues while staying home and caring for your mother. I love how this works, and here's my first quote... "By blessing others, your life will be blessed in the process."

To Hazel Payne and Steve Buckley. Thank you for our many years of friendship and for your great example of courage in following your dreams. Your success in the music business is testimony that when you plan and execute repeatedly, you will reach your goals.

And to the many others in my life who have played a part in my success journey, you know who you are.

Thank you, I love you all*

Sparkle C. Duncan

INTRODUCTION

I wrote this little book hoping that it falls into the hands of someone who really needs it, and possibly save a life. It appears that I'm beginning to attend two to three funerals a year of people who have died from lifestyle driven diseases. Everyone around me is on medications while others are having needless surgeries or dieing from so-called incurable diseases. I'm sure there are people out there searching for answers to their health problems. A lot more don't believe there's anything that can be done about their situation. I've met quite a few who just don't care anymore. They're doing things to their own bodies that they know is contributing to their demise.

This book is not for that last group of people. Those people wouldn't read a book like this or even touch it. For those of you who *are* searching, this book has reached your hands for a reason and the answers are simple. There are indeed things that you can do yourself to help your body get well. Although it's easy to do, the problem is that it's also easy not to do. The way a person gets well is that they make a decision to get well. When a person decides to do something, it's like homicide or suicide... they move forward and kill any notion of retreat. We have been so numbed down by the things we put into our bodies that we are unable to think clearly anymore. And we've been brainwashed to believe that we're not smart enough to figure anything out on our own.

Healing begins in the mind. True and permanent change cannot be accomplished until there is a change of mind, a complete paradigm shift. This book was written to let you (or someone that you love very much) know that there are answers, and the answers are simple, and simple is a good thing. Doctors may tell you differently but they are only going by what they've been taught. Once you make the decision to get yourself well and begin seeking out the answers, the answers will come. As you begin your journey, your mind will become less foggy and things will become clear. This simple book was written to wake you up and point you in the right direction. The rest is up to you. Your journey to wellness can begin today, just take the first step*

Sparkle C. Duncan

#1

Poor Health Is Reversible

Ok so you're under the notion that it's your destiny to be overweight, a diabetic, a chronic pain sufferer or be plagued with some disease for as long as you are alive. Honey, that couldn't be farther from the truth. You could at least be doing a whole lot better than you are now if you knew the truth about disease.

This is the problem; most people already

know that there may be something that they are doing or not doing that's contributing to their illness. Yep, that's right. Most of us are responsible for our own ill health yet we want to blame external circumstances and even God for our issues. We trash and tear down our bodies and then run to a doctor expecting him to piece us back together like Humpty Dumpty. The doctors are fully aware that most people are not willing to take responsibility for their own healing. People want the doctors to get rid of the problem for them so the doctors attempt to get rid of the problem by cutting it out, burning it out or medicating it out. In doing so, they tend to cause more problems than good.

You are responsible for your own healing. Not the doctors, not God, you! I believe pain and illness are blessings from God to let you know that something is wrong and you need to find out what the cause is and fix it. Usually we are causing our own problem. If we can find out what that is, we can stop doing it and get well. You can begin turning your situation around right now if you want. You can at least begin living a better quality of life than you've been living. You have to first get past the reality that you've messed up. That's ok because we all mess up. It's a part of the human experience, we are not perfect beings and we are going to mess up. We are also expected to live, learn and grow.

Imagine the unfortunate situation you would be in now if you never chose to learn to walk as a toddler even though you were fully capable. Good health is a choice. Do you choose to take your first steps towards getting yourself well and strong and looking great? Or do you choose to continue with the same old negative beliefs that do not support you? Even if you have a condition that you feel can never be healed, you can at least make your situation a lot better if you are willing to try something different. Most people won't even try something if they view it to be too simplistic to actually work.

I was told of a story about a famous tennis

player who had AIDS. He believed that his situation was terminal, there was no cure and that he would eventually die of his disease. Well this man was led (we are generally given answers but it's up to us to accept them) to the truth that he could be healed of his AIDS. In fact, he found a place where people were being healed from this so-called incurable disease. He even personally met some of the people who were being treated and healed. They let him read their charts that showed how sick they were before being treated and are now getting better. But this man's belief system was so firmly implanted that it would not allow him to believe what he was actually seeing with his own eyes.

Instead of going in for treatment for himself, he just kept going around asking the patients questions in disbelief that this *simple* method of healing was actually working without medications. One of the patients began yelling at him saying, "Man, look at me! I would have died by now if I didn't at least give this a try. Look at me, I'm being healed! You saw my charts showing how sick I was before these treatments! What is your problem?" The tennis player's strong belief system just would not allow him to believe what he was seeing. He refused to go in for treatment and unfortunately expired from his disease.

Understand this, old belief systems take a while to let go of for most people, and healing is not an overnight occurrence. It's taken years to get yourself in the position that you currently find yourself in, and it's going to take a while to turn it around. It's going to take work and it will require a lifestyle change. You're going to have to be willing to give up your old ways of doing things and adapt the "Sparkle Lifestyle". The Sparkle Lifestyle is a lifestyle that will clean you and heal you from the inside out. It will be even more rewarding because you will be the one that healed you, not the doctors. Yes, that's right. You are going to heal yourself!

If you're ready to make a change in your thinking and actions, if you're ready to put the work in and possibly give up some of the destructive habits that are making you ill, then I'm willing to share some secrets with you that will change your life. But if you're just going to keep holding on to the same old lame excuses like, "I'm big boned," or "it's in my genes," or "my uncle lived like this all his life and he lived to be 80 years old," or "that's the way I am," or "I can't," or "But I just love donuts," or whatever, then you should put this book down right now and keep on doing what you've been doing.

If you plan to continuing living the way you've been living but expecting a different result, then you know that's the definition of insanity so you may as well stop reading this now because you're wasting your time. You'll probably not finish reading it and you won't do the suggestions in it even if you do read it. So if you're not serious, then just throw this book in the trash or pass it on to someone who is.

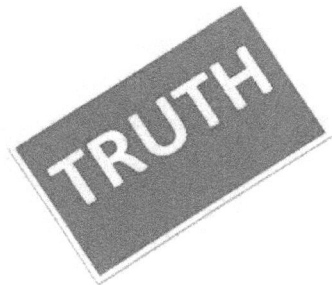

#2

Your Family History Does Not Necessarily Dictate Your Health Future

I know I may have sounded a bit harsh at the end of the previous chapter, but I wrote this book because I'm tired of attending funerals of family members and friends who pass away from preventable illnesses especially when they still had plenty of life left. So many people die in our country due to lack of knowledge and that is the reason I'm writing this little book. I want to at least spread awareness that these premature deaths are preventable.

The truth begins with the realization that we are responsible for our own health destruction and that we are also responsible for repairing it. I will attempt to guide you toward wellness, giving you some answers and resources to get you moving in the right direction. It's up to you to keep moving forward and not look back. Before you know it, you will be looking in the mirror at a whole new beautiful person.

You've probably heard this before and it's true for the most part, "If you want to be successful in life, look around you and take note of what everyone else is doing and then do the opposite." Take a moment and Google the following, "How many people die of cancer each year?" I Googled it a while back, and this is what came up: "According to the American Cancer Society's Global Cancer Facts and Figures, there were an estimated 7.5 million people who died from cancer in 2007." Here is another quote from Nanomedicalcenter.com posted February 1, 2010 ... "While cancer death statistics can vary from place to place it is generally estimated that roughly 7.2 to 7.5 million people worldwide die from cancer each year. In the United States alone where cancer death statistics are highly monitored, each year has seen a steady death rate of 550,000 to 600,000 people year after year, or roughly 1,500 people per day. This puts cancer as the second leading cause of death in the US just behind heart disease..."

So my question to you is this, if that many people are dying of cancer in the United States alone, don't you think it's wise for us to wake up, take notice of the American lifestyle and do something different? Understand this; disease isn't something that just randomly happens to some people. You don't catch a disease. A person can't just sneeze on you and you catch cancer or a heart attack or diabetes. Most diseases are lifestyle driven. It's time we take our heads out of the sand and see what's going on. It doesn't take much research to stumble upon the truth. We now have the almighty Internet and the controllers out there have not yet found a way to block its flow of free information. But I'm sure they're working on it.

We've been lied to folks, for a very long time. During my research over the years, I've met several people personally who have healed themselves of so-called incurable diseases. There are literally thousands more who have done the same. Why hasn't this info been made public? I won't go into that because it's easy to figure out once you realize that big pharmaceutical companies have been making **trillions** of dollars on the sale of medicines for years, and when you know that it's the large companies that generally donate the largest amount of money to the politicians.

I'll leave that for you to chew on for a

minute. I wouldn't advise you to do any investigation on that subject because it'll only disappoint you, hurt your feelings and make you angry. Especially if you actually meet, as I did, some of the alternative doctors who were healing people without the use of drugs only to have their clinics shut down and themselves thrown in jail. Did you know that a doctor can have his license revoked if he claims to **cure** someone of an incurable disease or uses the word **cure** for anything that is not a patented pharmaceutical? Shall I go on? Oh you don't believe me? Then check it out for yourself; I'm moving on.

Basically the reason we're sick and way overweight is due to our lifestyle and our environment. Our parents' contribution to us being ill is not necessarily their genes, but more so their health habits that we model. Our lifestyle is one of little movement and over indulgence of the wrong substances. Our environment is saturated with toxins and poisons to the point that it's a wonder anyone is still alive. The only reason we're still alive is that our bodies are constantly fighting day and night to keep us alive no matter what we do to it. If we would just give our bodies a little help, it wouldn't have to work so hard. We're ill because our bodies are overwhelmed with the crap that enters into it through the holes in our bodies i.e. the mouth, nose and skin.

The following is some basic scientific information that you need to be aware of in order to help you understand how it's possible to reverse the decline of your health and become well. In case you didn't know it, obesity is considered an illness too.

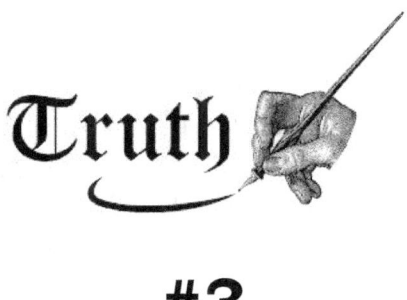

#3

Your Body Can Heal Itself

Although you can't see it or feel it, your organs are continuously working to keep you alive and well. You are wonderfully and marvelously made. Each cell in your body was designed to do a job and they all know exactly what to do. You have cells that carry nutrients to tissues and organs, other cells go through the body searching for invaders that may harm the body. The macrophage cell actually looks like it has an arm that reaches out and grabs the intruder and puts it into the lymphatic system and is eventually carried out of the body.

Cells eat like you do and also excrete waste materials just like you do. Other cells collect the waste material and dispose of it. Yes your cells are alive and they have jobs to do. New cells are created, they do their job and then they die. Let's look at the skin cells. New cells are formed at the bottom of the epidermis and takes about two weeks to one month to move from the bottom of the epidermis to the top. The older cells near the top die and are pushed to the surface. The surface of your skin is really dead skin cells.

The liver can regenerate itself. A part of your liver can be removed and put into another person's body and it will grow to normal size within a couple of weeks. It only takes a few days for bone marrow to regenerate.

The body is highly intelligent. One day I almost cut my thumb off while cutting onions with a very sharp knife. The knife crunched through my thumb nail and halfway through my thumb. My initial reaction was to rush myself to emergency but instead I decided that I wanted to watch my body heal itself. I threw my thumb into my mouth and pushed down really hard with my tongue to try to stop the bleeding and throbbing pain. Then I ran into the bathroom to find the Betadine and bandages. I opened the Betadine bottle and unwrapped the bandage with one hand. My injured thumb was still in my mouth with pressure being applied to it.

When I was ready, I quickly took my thumb out of my mouth. I didn't want to look at it because blood was oozing out fast. I poured a great deal of Betadine all over it, bandaged it up with a couple of bandages nice and snug. I saw the bandage fill up with blood but the blood did not ooze out so I figured I may be ok. I waited about six or seven days before removing the bandage. The blood had coagulated and there was a separation in the nail so I put more Betadine on it and covered it back snugly with a new bandage.

I changed the bandage every few days watching the healing process making sure I was only eating good food to help keep my body strong and healthy. My finger began to heal itself from the inside out. I watched as the skin on both sides of the nail healed completely, as well as the area under the nail. I also watched the crack on the surface of the nail grow forward until it grew completely out and I was able to trim it off.

Wow, that was so cool! I have a perfect looking thumb again. You cannot tell that it was ever injured! My body knew exactly what to do to heal itself. I didn't have to even think about it. I didn't say, "HEY RED BLOOD CELLS! COAGULATE AND STOP THE BLEEDING! HEY, HEY, YOU WHITE BLOOD CELLS! GET OVER HERE AND CLEAN UP ANY GERMS TO PREVENT INFECTION! HEY SKIN! MAKE

ME SOME NEW SKIN CELLS AND COVER UP THAT CUT! HEY YOU COME OVER HERE, AND YOU GO OVER THERE!!! No, all I had to do was just relax and observe. My body already knew what to do. I helped it out with a little antiseptic and covered it to keep the dirt out. My highly intelligent body did the rest on its own.

So what does that tell you? If your body is smart enough to grow new cells, is it smart enough to protect itself from deadly diseases? And if a disease has taken over the body, can the body still rid itself of the disease? The answer is it absolutely can, provided the person doesn't wait too late. So why are so many of us contracting diseases and dying from them? Read on.

Sparkle C. Duncan

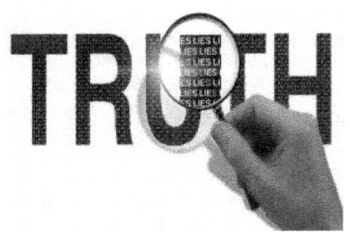

#4

The Cause of Disease

All of the diseases that I have studied were found to be caused by toxic environments both inside and out. Our bodies were not designed to live in toxicity. In biblical days people lived for hundreds of years. That was possible because their environment was clean and pure. Our bodies are being grossly overwhelmed with pollutants and toxins that our forefathers never had to deal with. I'll name a few:

- food additives

- chemical agriculture

- fluoride

- chlorine

- drugs

- altered GMO foods

- alcohol and nicotine

- immunization or vaccination

- cosmetics

- stress

- electronic fields.

It's called toxic overload and it's the reason we're ill.

This is the basic hidden information that I want to share with you. The human body was designed to heal itself. That may sound strange to some reading this material but if you go back and study your biology you'll find that to be true. So it's really not hidden information; it's just not talked about. It's considered hidden by the fact that most doctors normally don't share this information with their patients.

One doctor and I were discussing this topic and I asked him why he doesn't educate his patients. His answer is that most people aren't interested in hearing about healing themselves. They just want a quick fix in the form of a little pill. The problem with the little pill is that it merely masks the problem so the patient doesn't notice it. It also causes more toxicity and new symptoms. This doctor said that he does talk to his patients about a lifestyle change only when they're ready to listen. Sadly that's usually when it's too late.

If you've never driven a car before, you will need to know how it works before you get behind the wheel so you won't kill yourself or tear up the car right?. The same goes for your body, if you don't know how it works, you will probably wreck it like the majority of us are doing now. This is how it works:

The Heart
The heart pumps blood throughout the body. The blood nourishes the tissues

and organs so that they can do what they were designed to do. When the organs are living in a toxic environment, they become sick and unable to do their job. The main job of the cells and organs of your body is to keep you alive.

The Liver

The liver is designed to convert toxic products into nontoxic ones, it actively participates in metabolism of Carbohydrates, Fats, Proteins, Vitamins and Minerals, it excretes bile pigments, bile salts, cholesterol through bile and it synthesizes plasma proteins. The liver is so important that it is the only organ that can fully regenerate itself within two weeks or less. If the liver is not working, it cannot rid the body of harmful toxins that will surely kill you if not disposed of.

The Kidneys

The kidneys perform the essential function of removing waste products from the blood and regulating the water fluid levels. It produces hormones and absorbs minerals. When the kidneys aren't functioning properly, the blood becomes filthy and parasites can actually be seen floating around in the blood. The blood cells become deformed and disease sets in.

The Pancreas

The pancreas makes enzymes and hormones such as insulin and glucagon for the body. Enzymes are necessary for the digestion of food. The lack of enzymes is one reason for obesity. When the pancreas is weak and sick, it can't produce enzymes so we need to get it from our food. When we eat dead foods that lack nutrients and enzymes, we tend to overeat because our bodies crave real food but that's not what its getting. No enzymes, no digestion, more hunger, more fake food and the cycle continues. We become obese in the process but continue the cycle because the fast foods are addictive. Abnormal hormone and insulin levels cause other dangerous health issues as well.

The Stomach

The stomach dumps food into the small intestine. The primary function of the **small intestine** is the absorption of nutrients and minerals found in food, and it is followed by the large intestine.

The main function of the **large intestine**, also called the **colon**, is to transport waste/toxins out of the body and to absorb water from the waste before it leaves. When waste first reaches the large intestine, it dumps into it like sludge from a chute. The sludge solidifies as it travels through the large intestine. If all is well, the waste is in solid form (but not too solid) when it reaches the rectum.

It is believed that most disease begins in the colon. If the colon is cleansed on a regular basis, then most disease would not be created. Unfortunately, most Americans are constipated which allows waste material to sit in the colon causing it to become diseased. When that happens, the intestine begins to leak toxins into the blood stream causing disease to settle into other areas of the body. A great deal of Americans, men and women alike, are walking around looking pregnant when in reality they are literally just full of crap!

One particular naturopathic doctor spoke of people coming into his clinic with serious illnesses. His first step in healing them was to get their gut cleaned. One guy lost over 30 pounds and his symptoms disappeared. The same has happened for others who were overweight. After simply going through a detox program most people lost 20 to 30 pounds. Doctors trained in western methods instead, cut out the diseased colon, sometimes very large amounts of it, which of course hinders the digestion process. This is very upsetting to me because once the colon is clean, it will begin to repair its own damage. I advocate giving the body a chance to repair itself except in *immediate* life-threatening situations.

As I mentioned earlier, toxins found in our environment both inside and outside of us are the reason we die prematurely because they breakdown the body's defenses. The body is designed to heal itself by continually ridding itself of harmful toxins. The problem is we are unnaturally being bombarded with way more toxins than our bodies are able to get rid of. Yet it comes up with some pretty incredible ways of protecting itself in order to give us a few more years of life.

For example, your body is constantly trying to keep itself balanced between the acidic and the alkaline levels. If your body is too acidic, you will die. If it becomes too alkaline you will also die. Your blood should be ideally at a 7.6 PH balance, just a little alkaline. But most people are way on the acidic side of the chart. Think about it, what does acid do to steel? It eats holes in it. Acid in your body will eat holes in teeth too. FYI, sugar on teeth is not what causes cavities, sugar converts into acid and it's the acid that eats holes in teeth. If acid will eat holes in bone and steel, what do you think it will do to your arteries?

Your highly intelligent cells understand what will happen, so if we don't stop putting things into our body like sodas, sugar and processed foods that cause the body to become acidic, then the body will do what it has to do to protect itself. Your body will produce calcium or take it from your bones and line your arteries with it so that you won't bleed out and die. The problem with that is now you have a disease called hardening of the arteries which blocks the blood flow.

My mother was found to have five brain aneurysms which were serviced with platinum coils. She was given a blood thinner so that the blood can flow more freely through her clogged blood vessels but a year later a piece of plaque was believed to have broken off causing her to suffer a massive stroke. My mother is a very strong woman because fifteen years later, she's still here.

Sparkle C. Duncan

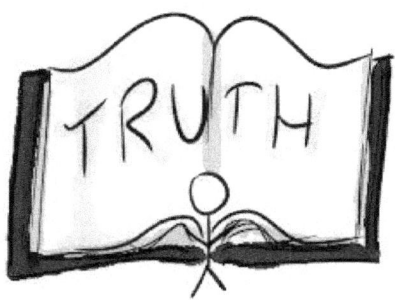

#5

True Healing Does Not Mean Going On Another Diet

Ok, now's the time to make a decision. Do you really want to be healthy or will you chose to continue your slow decline, until you're six feet under? True healing does not mean going on another diet. True lasting healing begins with a **paradigm shift**. You are going to have to be willing to change the way you think before taking

43

action or your actions will be futile. Diets don't work because first of all, most of them are unhealthy, and second of all once you are done you will go back to doing the same things that made you ill in the first place.

Many people have tried numerous times to lose weight but have been unsuccessful. There are reasons why. One reason is, again because their food choices create acid in their bodies. Normally the body is able to remove the acids in small amounts. But when its coming in faster than the body can get rid of it, the body will store the acid in the fat tissues to protect itself. When you're acidic as most people are in this country, your body will hold on to the fat no matter how hard you try to get rid of it in order to protect your arteries. The proper way to lose weight is to create more alkalinity in your body instead of acid by consuming more raw green foods. When your body is in the proper PH balance for a while meaning no more acid overflow, it will realize that the danger is gone then begin letting go of the fat.

A lifestyle change is the only answer to lasting weight loss and good health. Be patient with yourself in your quest for good health. Slow and steady wins the race, so take your time with it and enjoy the journey.

I want you to experience what life can be like when you're healthy and disease free! It may mean that you will have to give up some of your comfort foods but I'm telling you, **nothing** tastes as good as good health feels! Besides you can adapt some new comfort foods that taste great and are healing to your body.

Again, please do not take drastic steps with your healing (unless you are dying) because you will probably fail. Instead start with small baby steps and step your way to success. If you stick with your healing program long enough, you won't want to go back to doing the things that were killing you.

When you begin to shed those extra deadly pounds and begin putting into your body the things that will heal your cells and tissues and give you an unlimited supply of energy, you won't want to stop your new lifestyle. But be careful, the new energy may cause you to do crazy things like jump on a bike and race your kids around the block, take your son's skate board and try to do what he's doing or challenge some high school youngster to a slam-dunk contest. Listen, the energy may be there but not the skill. So take it easy or you may end up in the hospital for other reasons.

Just think how your life will change when you're healthy. Think how the relationships with your loved ones will change for the better. Think of the new energy you will have to help you deal with all the day-to-day stress and to enable you to get more done in a day. If you have a demanding job, your energy levels won't crash before you get home leaving nothing for your family. If you have been sick or overweight for a long time, getting well will make you feel like you're having an out-of-body experience. You *will* be out of your body. You will have traded the old one for a new and improved model. It won't be a dream. It'll be a real experience and **you** will have created it! You'll take full credit and it will feel incredible!

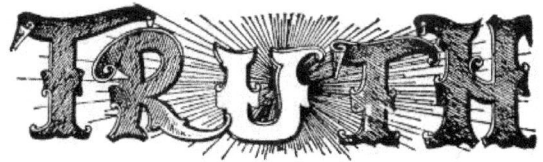

#6

True Health Secrets From Our Ancestors

What I'm about to share with you is called a lifestyle change. I'm going to share the secrets of our ancestors—things that were "no brainers" to them, because they didn't have any alternative except to follow God's perfect design. When we were created, we were given everything we needed to sustain a long, healthy life. Just like there are laws for science with a cause-and-effect, like the law of gravity, whatever goes up must come down, there are also health laws that when broken will create a negative effect.

Our culture totally ignores the laws of health because we've created a fast-paced generation. Everyone wants results without putting in any effort. That's not how it works. The law of planting and reaping goes like this ... if you want to reap a harvest you must first plant a seed. Good health does not just come by osmosis. It's going to take some work. If you're lazy and don't want to work for what you want, you will never achieve success. It's going to take planning and commitment.

While I was in school, I took an anthropology class and we studied a couple of groups of primitive people. Primitive man lived an entirely different lifestyle than we do now, and they did not suffer with high blood pressure, strokes, heart attacks, diabetes, Parkinson's disease or any of the illnesses that we suffer with today.

The African Bushmen were discovered not many years ago and when tested, were found to be totally healthy. No disease at all, not even one case of obesity found among them. The documentaries that we watched showed that these people lived a whole lot differently than we do. They had no refrigerators or microwaves so they ate most of their food raw. There were no pesticides sprayed on the foods that they consumed. No artificial colors, dyes, antibiotics or preservatives were added. Their food was not processed or tampered with in any way. It was all live, organic and perfect—just the way God made it and designed for us to consume.

God made real food, the type of food that our cells understand. But man wants to tamper with that perfect food by taking it apart, removing stuff from it and adding things to it in order to benefit their bottom line. The greed of man is causing our demise. If we don't get a grip, not only will our bodies continue to deteriorate, but our planet as well and there will be no reversal.

Back to primitive man, they had no

automobiles or other pollutants. They were always out in the healing sun and fresh air and they were always moving with their **feet touching the earth**. You electricians out there know about grounding. Our bodies have a great deal of electricity in them and need to be grounded just like the electrical equipment in our homes because our cells have electric fields in them too. The soles of our shoes today are usually made of rubber. Because our feet rarely touch the earth anymore, we are subject to many health imbalances. But that's another teaching as well. Primitive man didn't have cars so they walked everywhere they went. Asians say that one should walk five thousand steps a day for our good health. I say ten thousand.

I asked a friend of mine how he lost over 350 pounds. He said he just walked his fool head off. He walked every morning before going to work, during his lunch break and in the evening when he got home. Now to maintain his weight, he walks every day at work during his lunch break.

Back to the Bushmen, they also ate very little meat. Most of their food consisted of vegetables, roots, fruits, nuts, seeds and berries. The little meat that they did eat was clean, meaning the animals were healthy, roaming freely, eating organic vegetation, not ground up animal by-products. There were no parasites in the meat and they were not pumped with antibiotics and hormones. The Bushmen's food, water and air environment was clean and pure, thus their bodies were easily able to function normally which equated to no disease forming in their bodies. Their lifestyle was very simple. Ours is complicated and stressful. Oh by the way, stress is a major cause of disease today.

One of our modern men tried to explain to a bushman the notion of ownership. The bushman could not comprehend what he was saying since they believe that everything belongs to the gods, including the earth and land. So how can a man pay another man for land? Everyone had access to the same things...wood, leaves, stones... if a child wanted a toy just like his friend, he would just go out and find some sticks to make his own toy. There weren't many reasons for fighting or jealousy. No one among them had any bills to pay. They just lived life and enjoyed each others company. What a simple culture.

But we Americans don't like simple. We want to complicate everything and create a lot of unnecessary drama in our life. It's time to stop the negative toxic cycle we've created for ourselves—time to try something different. How about getting back to the basics and sticking with what works.

#7

Your Healing Can Begin Today

Trying to implement simple strategies in our fast-paced, complicated lives may be a bit challenging but it's doable. It will take some effort at first but will become easy over time. Old habits are hard to break and it takes about 30 days to create a new one. It'll be worth it in the long run. Are you still with me? I guess you're serious ... then let's begin.

The first thing you want to do is start eliminating as many toxins as you possibly can from your outside environment. Next you're going to begin eliminating the toxins that you've been putting inside your body. But not to overwhelm you, let's start with baby steps.

1. *Eliminate outside environmental toxins:*

I try to do some form of exercise every day or at least five days a week. One day I decided to exercise my face muscles to keep my face looking young and healthy. As I was opening my mouth wide and closing it and switching my lips from side to side, I noticed that the inside of my mouth was a little tighter on one side. So while looking in the mirror, I opened my mouth wide and saw a small gray spot on the inside of my cheek way back in the back of my mouth. I kept an eye on it for a couple of weeks to see if it would grow. Yes it was growing.

My dentist ordered a biopsy. The results were Abnormal Basil Cells, which was a breakdown of cells in the wall of my cheek and a 15% chance that it could grow into cancer. I asked what could have **caused** it (most people don't ask that question). I didn't just want to get rid of the problem; I also wanted to know what may have caused it so that it won't happen again. I figured if I could get rid of the **cause**, then I could focus on getting rid of the disease.

I was given a list of possible causes. One of the things on the list was EMF signals. EMF stands for Electric Magnetic Fields. Some of the things that emit electric magnetic fields (radiation) are televisions, lamps, radios, refrigerators, micro waves, computers, cell phones and those cell phone towers that they have erected almost everywhere.

After thinking about it for a while, I realized that I had been holding my cell phone up to my face in that same spot every day for hours as I was making calls to prospective clients for a business that I was working on. I was also under a great deal of personal stress at that time and sitting in front of my computer constantly. Once I figured out the possible cause, I stopped putting my cell phone up to my head and purchased one of those blue tooth gadgets.

I thought I had found a great solution for making my calls without putting my phone up to my head. Well as I studied more about how to heal myself of the basil cells, I found that the blue tooth ear piece may cause brain cancer. I only had my blue tooth for a couple of weeks and then threw it in the garbage. I could have sold it but I felt like I would be selling someone cancer. I didn't feel good about that idea so I just tossed it.

Look around and take note of all the radio masts that are being erected everywhere to service all the millions of cell phones in our world. Many of them are camouflaged by fake pine trees. Look around in your area to see where they're located and try to limit your exposure to them. EMF causes sleep disturbances, headaches, skin rashes, heart palpitations, vertigo and cancer.

There are screens that you can purchase for your computers to reduce the EMF exposure. There is also grounding tools for your body that can be used for your protection. Purchase good earphone buds that connect to your cell phone, then place your cell phone at least six inches away from your body. Turn it off when you're not using it and try not to carry it on your body even if it's in the off position. Turn off all electronic devices especially if they are around you when you sleep at night.

Your home may be full of toxins. Paint is one of the largest offenders. The older paints can be extremely hazardous to your body. If you live in a house that was built before 1970, then it was most likely painted with lead-based paint.

A quote from Dr. Edward Group: "Toxic mercury was also added to latex paints until around the 1990. Today's paints have VOCs added to them which stands for Volatile Organic Compounds. They are used to make the paint dry faster but they are extremely toxic. Too much VOC build-up in the body can cause eye, nose and throat irritation, headaches, loss of coordination, nausea and damage to the liver, kidneys and central nervous system. VOCs have also been shown to cause cancer in animals." If you are going to paint your home, ask for environmentally safe/non-toxic paint options.

2. *Stress, the silent killer*

I was under so much stress at a time in my life that I developed an irregular heartbeat. One time the stress in my life was so elevated that when I laid down to sleep, I could feel my heart knocking around in my chest. I literally felt my body shake from side to side each time my heart beat. That was scary. Every time it happened, I noticed I was thinking about my stressful situation. I realized if I wanted to keep breathing, I needed to let it go. I had to remove myself from my stressful environment.

Sometimes you may have to make a decision to divorce yourself from people you love or die trying to change them. Sometimes, the best way to change another person's actions is to change your own. If you're married or having problems with a family member or friend and you've tried prayer, counseling, changing the way you react to that person, showing love instead of revenge, you've given it an adequate amount of time but still no change for the positive, then it's probably not God's will that you stay in that relationship. God is a God of peace. He is not the author of confusion or chaos. It is especially time to leave if the stress is greatly affecting your health and safety.

I once read a great article about stress management from a website called HelpGuide.org. Go there and click on "Stress." After reading that article, click on "Relaxation Techniques." There are a lot of good books, articles and DVDs out there that can assist you in dealing with stress. Whichever method you chose, please work with it because stress is being called "The Enemy Within" and it will take you out!

Our ancestors who lived among the wild animals occasionally were caught in fight-or-flight situations. Here is a quote from Charlotte Gerson, a natural healer: "In those stressful situations, heart rate increases, blood sugar levels rises, the pupils dilate to see better and the digestions slows down to divert energy to the limbs. Adrenaline and cortisol rush into the system. All these changes disappear when the situation is resolved either by fighting the enemy or fleeing to safety.

These days, the threats are mainly nonviolent and the challenges tend to cause frustration, simmering rage or repressed tension—all of which find no outlet. After all, we can't wrestle with a hypercritical boss or escape from a maddening traffic jam, so the organism stays in an unnaturally aroused state. Just like our cave-dwelling ancestors, modern people also go through the three phases of alarm, resistance and finally, exhaustion.

In due course, the stress-induced hormonal changes can lead to a wide range of diseases, including hypertension, coronary thrombosis, brain hemorrhage, gastric or duodenal ulcers, arteriosclerosis, arthritis, kidney disease and allergic reactions. Above all, the immune system is weakened and we know how dangerous that is."

Charlotte says that normally it's our reaction to stress that causes the illness more than the illness itself. People's normal reaction to stressors are to smoke more, drink more alcohol, put in more hours at work, live on junk food, take sleeping pills to fight insomnia and then more pills to face the new day, which all speeds up the decline in our health.

3. *Remove Internal Toxins*

Removing toxins inside of you is not difficult. You can start by eating foods that detoxify the body. Detox foods are the ones with the most chlorophyll. Those are your green vegetables like broccoli, spinach, lettuce, parsley and cilantro. Parsley and cilantro clean the blood. Additionally chia seeds, aloe vera, dandelion and lemon water clean the liver.

The best way to do a detox is to use a juicer and juice your veggies. That way you can get a lot more detoxifying foods inside you. Just eating your raw green foods is fine, but you will need to consume a lot in order to detox. Juicing greens alone does not taste very good so you may want to juice some sweet fruit with it and a little agave nectar or raw honey to make it palatable.

Drink immediately instead of refrigerating to get the most nutritional value. If you make a big batch, try to consume all of it that same day. It is advised to go on a seven-day juice fast or longer to get the maximum benefit. Juice fasting is also good because it gives your digestive system a rest and a chance to heal.

A great juicer to use for juicing both greens and fruits and that extract the most juice while leaving a dryer pulp is the Omega juicer. Chose any one of the 8004-8008 series. They are extremely durable, less noisy, easy to clean and it comes with a <u>15 year warranty</u>. The latest model is the NC800. It's a more expensive machine. It has a wider mouth so you can get larger pieces of fruits and veggies down the shoot at one time and it extracts a little more juice. Whatever juicer you chose to purchase is fine, just get one.

4. *Stop Polluting Your Body*

Continually putting poison foods into your body while you are trying to remove toxins is not getting you anywhere. Toxic foods are just about everything that is purchased at a major supermarket chain (although I understand some markets are stocking healthier options these days). Stay away from processed and refined foods like white sugar and white flour. Consume as much organic food as possible. Organic foods are clean foods that have not been tampered with. Do not eat foods that are loaded with chemicals. You will need to become a label reader. If you can't pronounce it or don't understand what it means then you probably don't want it in your body. For instance, read the ingredients on the back of the Quaker Oats oatmeal box. The ingredients say "Rolled Oats." That's it. It means that product is real food and may be consumed.

Again, I don't recommend that you go crazy with this all at once. Just become aware and begin making healthier choices. Do your shopping at the nearest *health food store* or *Farmers Market* for starters. You can find the nearest one to you on the internet by Googling it. (If you don't know what that means, just ask your kids).

That's pretty much it. I don't want to

overwhelm you with too much information in this book. This book was designed as a quick read to deliver some simple information to you. I just want you to know that good health is not only possible, it's possible for you! Your past health history or that of your family members does not necessarily dictate your future health. It does if you continue to do what they did. Good health is under your control and it's yours if you want it.

For more information on good health and how to achieve it, visit the following online sites. You may also contact me at the following email address.

Website:
www.thesparklelifestyle.com
Facebook:
www.facebook.com/thesparklelifestyle
Email:
sparkle@thesparklelifestyle.com

You must take action **now!**. The successful people in this world are the ones who take action as soon as the emotion hits. So get yourself locked in with a partner or company that is dedicated to helping you create a

"**Lifestyle Change**." Do not go for the quick-fix gimmicks. Instead, go for something that promotes lasting change.

Start today by choosing one easy, small step toward your good health like walk to the corner and back or drink one less soda each day. Again, make sure you lock arms with a partner or company that will come along side you and assist you with your health goals, someone to hold you accountable. Change is not easy, you're going to need some help.

May God bless you on your journey to good health! I hope to some day meet you and congratulate you in person on a job well done.

Until then, take care, God bless and...

Be Well *

Sparkle C. Duncan

ABOUT THE AUTHOR

Sparkle C. Duncan has inspired people of all ages to feel good about themselves and to reach for excellence in their lives. As a child, she remembers spending time with her grandmother and stopping to converse with senior citizens. She was drawn to seniors because they loved spending time with her and was willingly to shared their knowledge with her. From their answers to her questions she began to understand why some seniors lived long healthy lives and others were sick and in pain.

Sparkle continued to seek knowledge from books, developed a large in-home library and went on to earn a degree in communications and social Science from the University of Southern California.

Sparkle became a teacher and mentor to children in multiple school districts in southern California and is now teaching children and adults to create a body that is healthy and vibrant. She has found that good health is the foundation to a clear mind, vitality, longevity and tons of energy.